12 Perils of Pregnancy:

12 Little "Joys" of Pregnancy No Other Book Will Tell You!

by Michelle Zelinger

The contents of this work, including, but not limited to, the accuracy of events, people, and places depicted; opinions expressed; permission to use previously published materials included; and any advice given or actions advocated are solely the responsibility of the author, who assumes all liability for said work and indemnifies the publisher against any claims stemming from publication of the work.

All Rights Reserved
Copyright © 2020 by Michelle Zelinger

No part of this book may be reproduced or transmitted, downloaded, distributed, reverse engineered, or stored in or introduced into any information storage and retrieval system, in any form or by any means, including photocopying and recording, whether electronic or mechanical, now known or hereinafter invented without permission in writing from the publisher.

Dorrance Publishing Co
585 Alpha Drive
Suite 103
Pittsburgh, PA 15238
Visit our website at www.dorrancebookstore.com

ISBN: 978-1-6480-4018-4
eISBN: 978-1-6480-4028-3

12 Perils of Pregnancy:

*12 Little "Joys" of Pregnancy
No Other Book Will Tell You!*

About the Author:

    <u>12 Perils of Pregnancy</u> are actually 12 things that happened to my body during pregnancy. When I went to the doctors office and said, "blank is happening to my body . . . is this normal?" They would say, "yes." But, I wondered why I didn't find much about these symptoms in most of my reading. During my pregnancy I made a list as the days went on. Hence, <u>12 Perils of Pregnancy</u>. As much as women are different so are their prenatal symptoms. You may experience these 12 perils or you may not. These 12 perils may be real and difficult to experience, but humor can get you through the tough times. The final reward . . . is a beautiful precious child you can call yours. I dedicate this book to my daughter Jenelle Nicole, my son Dominic Ian, my mother, my mother's mother and her mother . . .

About the Artist:

    Jamz Lackner was a restless native of Colorado. He owned *Jamz Cardz*; where he originated and generated his own line of greeting cards. Jamz also painted, specializing in "residential portraiture". Jamz lived in Denver, Colorado. He was surrounded by a menagerie of creatures both human and non. Jamz lost his life to cancer at the age of forty.

Jamz David Lackner 1962-2002

Congratulations
on the arrival of
your new baby!

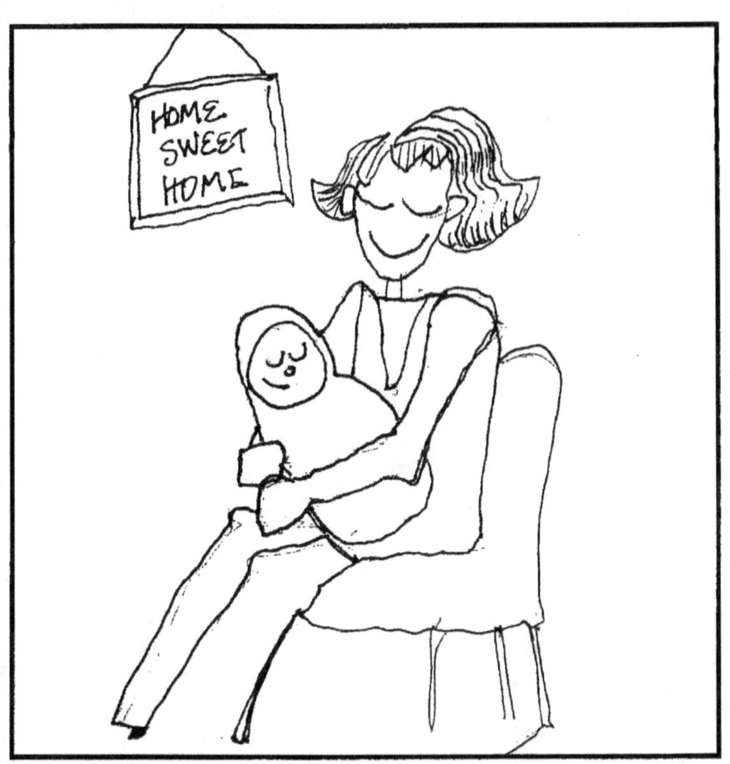

1. Soft Pelvis:

**Your pelvis is preparing for having a baby;
it softens to allow for vaginal delivery.
Your pelvis may feel like it is bruised.**

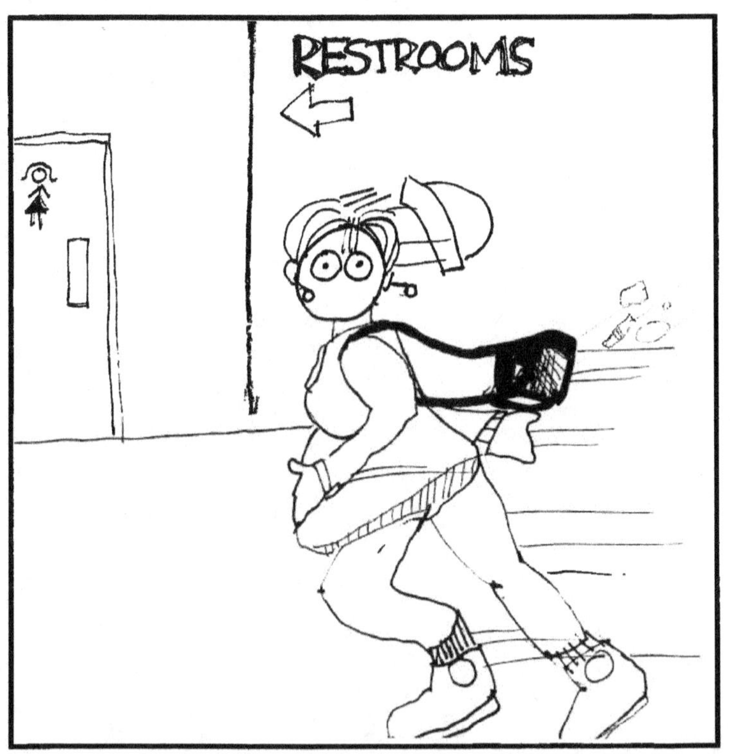

2. Loss of Bladder Control:
This is caused by an increased volume of body fluids and pressure from your growing uterus. Keep your eyes open for restroom stops!

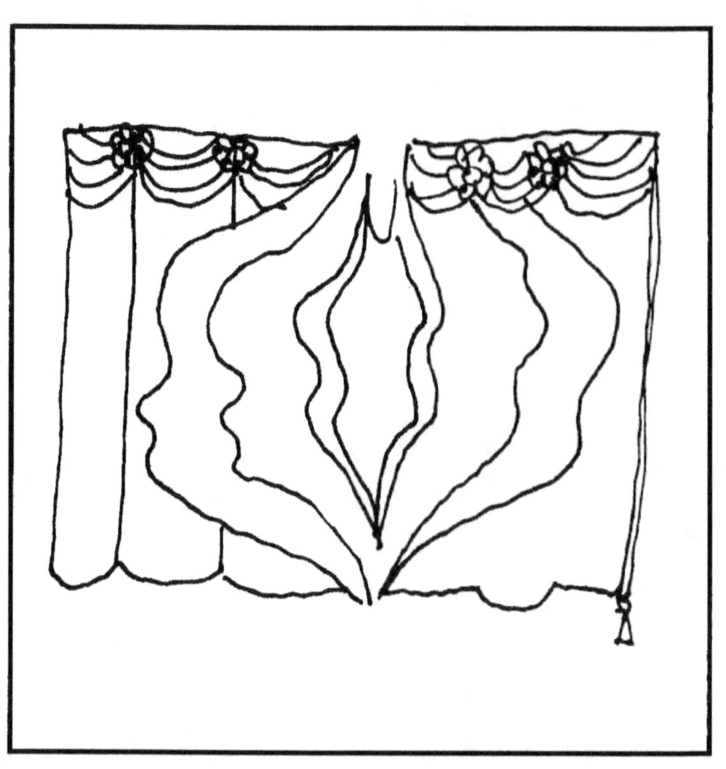

3. Enlarged Vagina and Labia:

Your vagina and labia may feel swollen; this is caused by an increased blood flow in the body. Don't worry, this is normal.

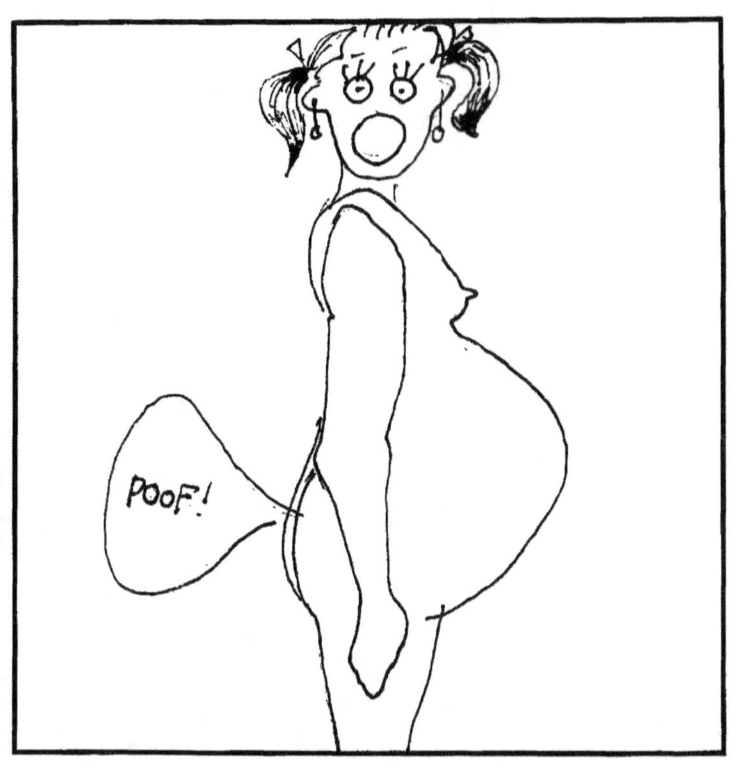

4. Gas:

**Intestinal distress; no explanation really.
Just let it rip.**

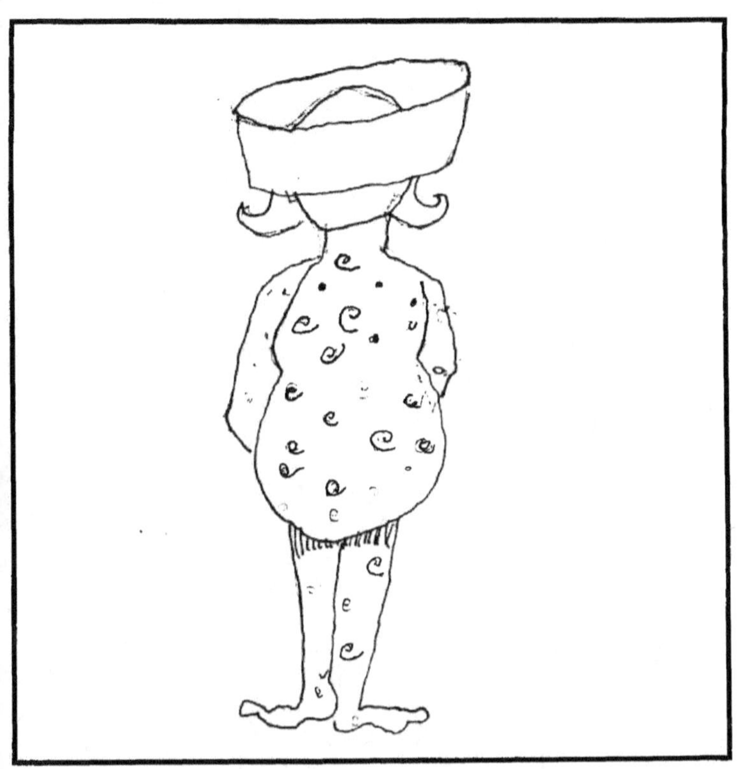

5. Rash:

An increase in perspiration comes from sweat glands and may cause heat rash. This will usually disappear after delivery.

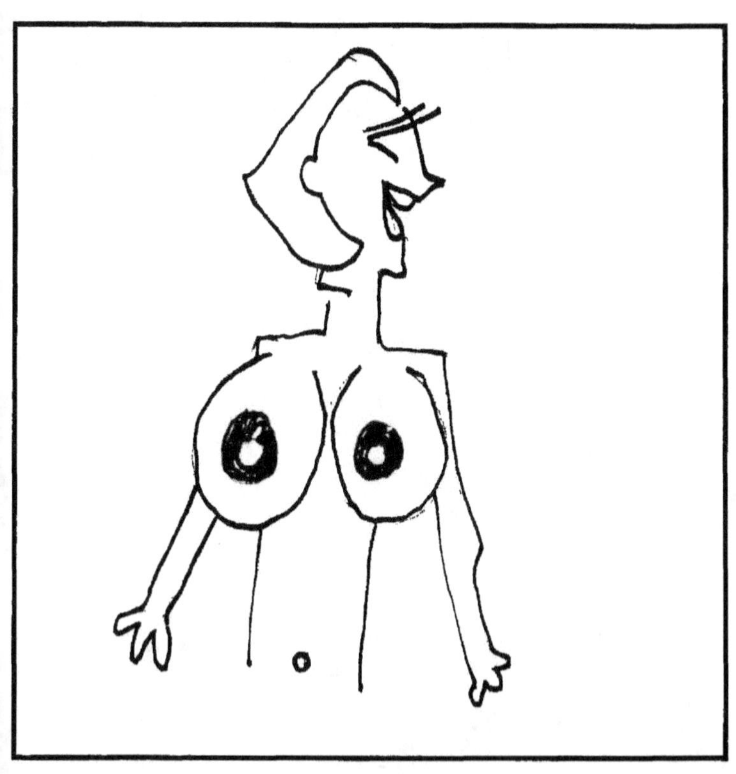

6. Darkened Areolas:

Breast changes are caused by increases in progesterone and estrogen; the pigmented area around the nipple may become darker.

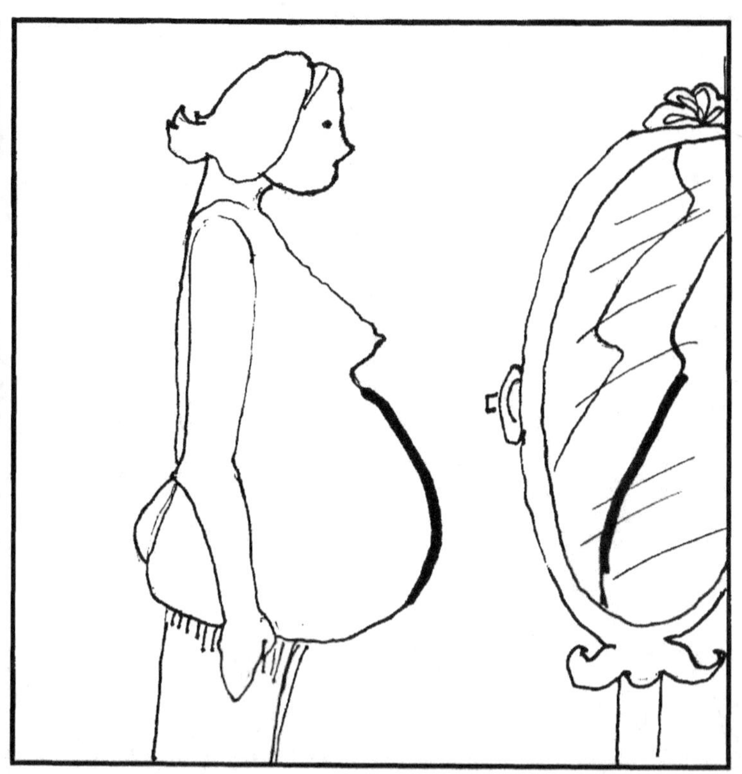

7. Linea Negra:

A dark line from the middle of your rib cage to your pubic bone. No one knows why you get it; you just do. This too will disappear after delivery.

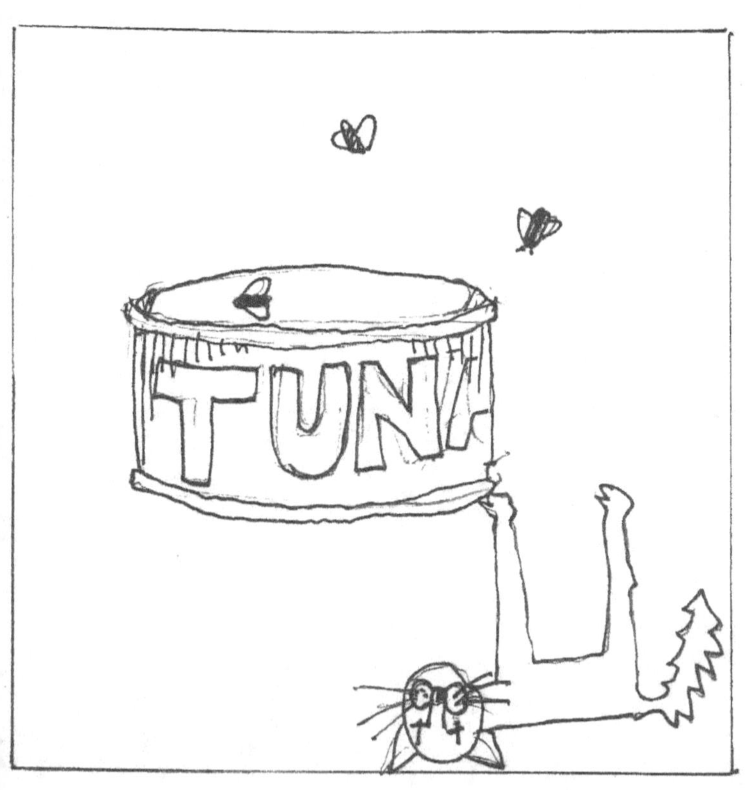

8. Increased Vaginal Odor:

This is a hormonal change. No matter how many showers you take your vagina won't come out smelling like roses.

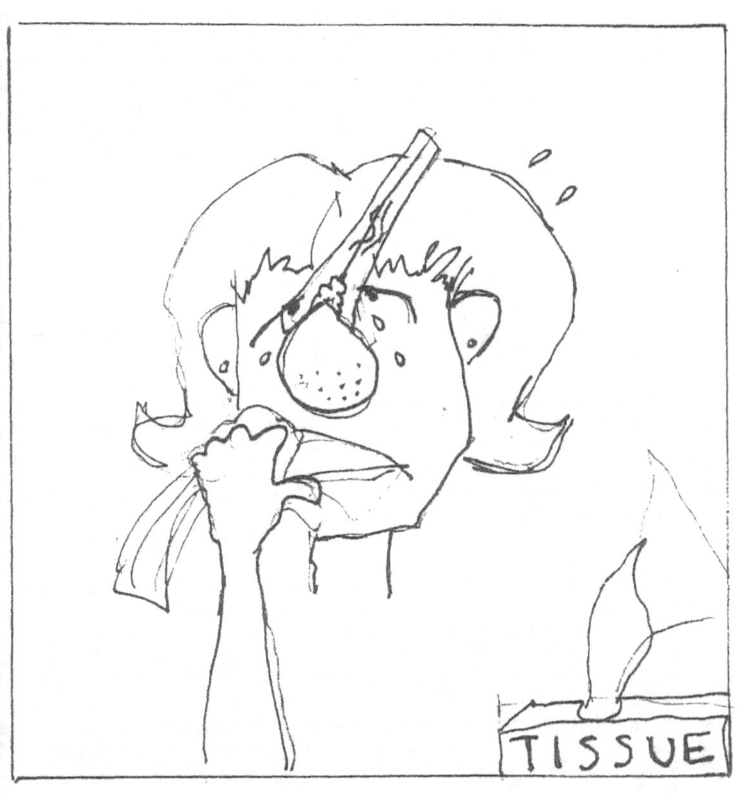

9. Clogged Sinus:

This is a result of hormonal changes. As estrogen increases, the swelling of blood vessels increases.

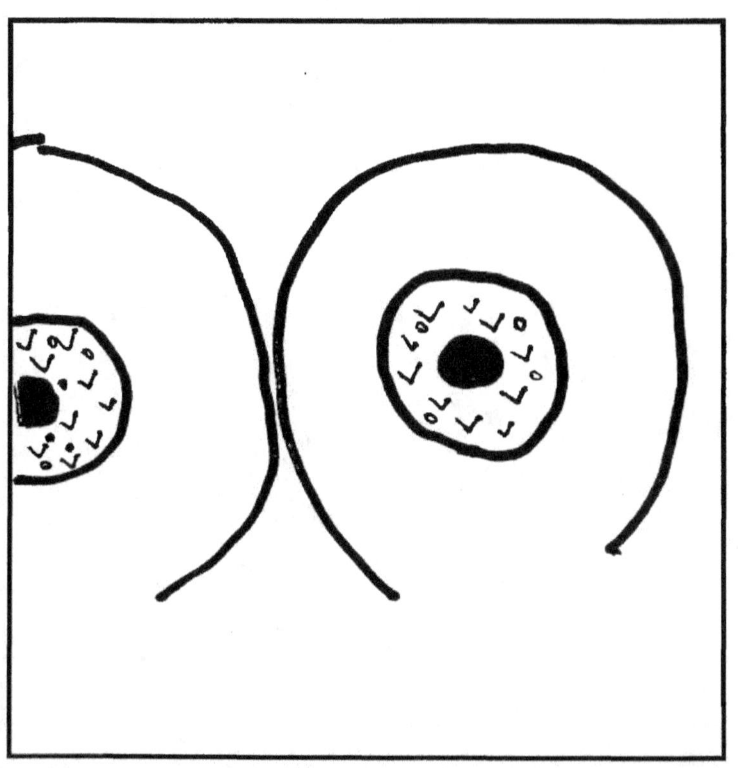

10. Areola Warts (Bumps):

These bumps are also called sweat glands. The little bumps on the areola may become more prominent during pregnancy.

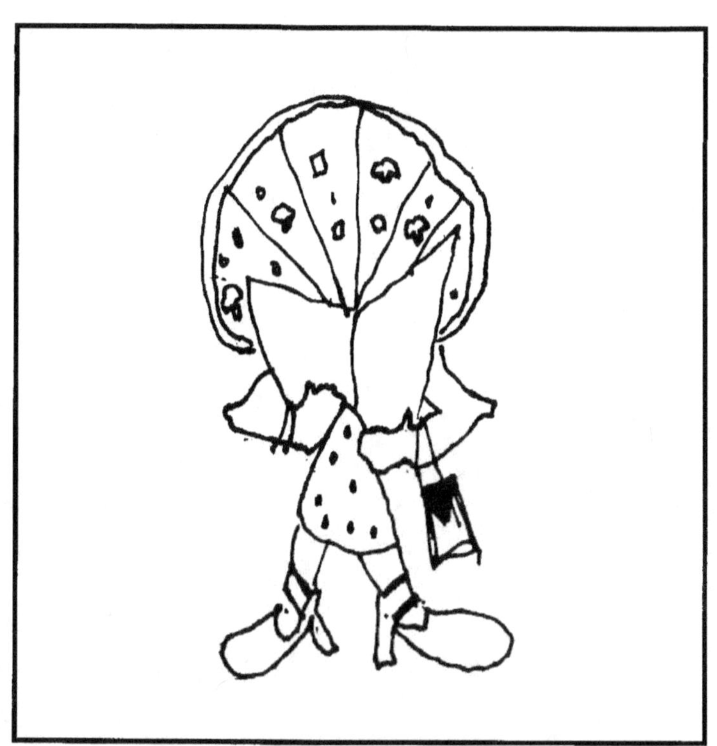

11. Acne

Hormonal changes can increase the secretion of oils in the skin. Drink plenty of water; it's one of the best pore-reducers around.

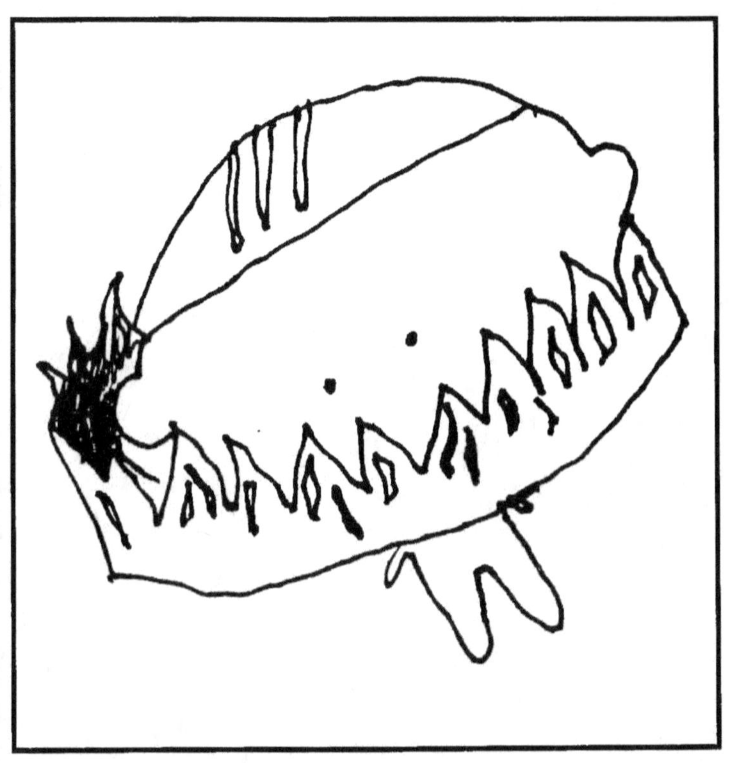

12. Ring of Fire

During delivery the vagina is being stretched, sometimes giving a burning sensation. Hence: Ring of Fire. Just do your best and push!

www.ingramcontent.com/pod-product-compliance
Lightning Source LLC
Chambersburg PA
CBHW050711250726
48662CB00002B/956